MARISSA HILL

How I Survived Death: My Battle with Postpartum Cardiomyopathy—The Silent Killer Every New Mother Needs to Know About.

Recognizing the Signs: What Every Woman Should Watch for After Childbirth That May Not Be Just Normal Postpartum Symptoms

Contents

How I Survived Death: My Battle with Postpartum Cardiomyopathy—The Silent Killer Every New Mother Needs to Know About.

Recognizing the Signs: What Every Woman Should Watch for After Childbirth That May Not Be Just Normal Postpartum Symptoms

2

Introduction

Bringing new life into the world is one of the most beautiful and transformative experiences a woman can go through. But what happens when the joy of motherhood is overshadowed by a silent, life-threatening condition? This is my story—a story of survival, strength, and the terrifying experience of facing death just three months after giving birth to my beautiful baby.

Postpartum cardiomyopathy is a rare yet deadly form of heart failure that can occur after childbirth. It's a silent killer, often masked by what we assume are the "normal" aches, pains, and body changes associated with postpartum recovery. But for many women, these subtle signs can mean something far more serious—and the difference between life and death lies in recognizing them.

In this book, I take you through my personal journey, from the joyful moments of welcoming my child into the world to the terrifying realization that my body was failing me. I will share the signs I missed, the ones I didn't understand, and the ones I hope every new mother will recognize before it's too late. This book is more than just my story—it's a guide. It's my way of raising awareness about postpartum cardiomyopathy, empowering women to recognize that what they're feeling might not be "just" postpartum fatigue.

My hope is that through my experience, I can help save lives. No woman should face the fear of losing her life after the joy of gaining a child. This is a wake-up call for all mothers, partners, and healthcare providers. Because sometimes, it's more than just motherhood—it's survival.

3

My Story

My beautiful baby boy was born in December, just three days after my birthday, making that time even more special. My birthday was on Christmas day, and my greatest gift was my son. I couldn't wait to meet him. I was nervous because his birth was a scheduled C-section due to my medical history. When he arrived, I was overwhelmed with happiness. However, it was a hard time to give birth due to the restrictions of the COVID-19 pandemic—only my spouse was able to visit.

Recovery after birth was brutal. C-sections are no joke, and this was my second one. I had some help at home, though not as much as I would've liked, but I was grateful. As mothers, we often push past the pain, focusing on our children. I had my sweet baby boy and my darling daughter to tend to, even though my body felt like it had been hit by an eighteen-wheeler. I kept going and eventually, the days got easier—or so I thought.

As I started to heal, I noticed something strange. I was getting breathless and exhausted while doing simple tasks. I would sweat profusely, even when I wasn't doing anything. At first, I brushed it off, thinking I was just naturally prone to sweating. But deep down, I knew something wasn't right.

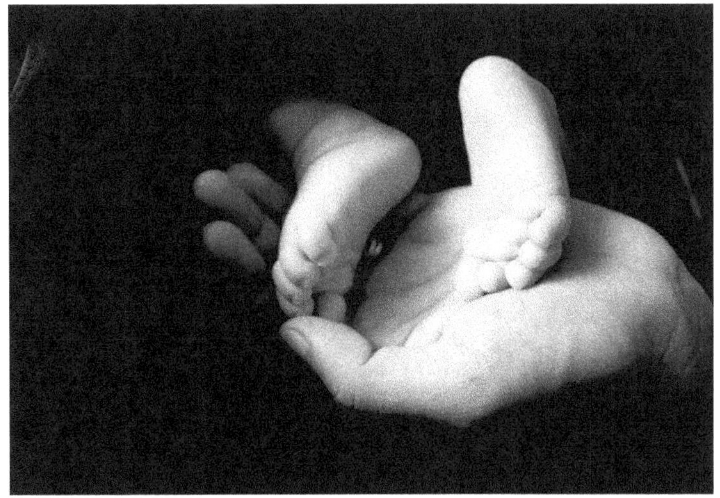

4

Recognizing the Signs

I vividly remember the time I gave birth to my daughter four years earlier. About a week after coming home from the hospital, I found myself gasping for air and struggling to breathe. Alarmed, I rushed to the emergency room, but the doctors were baffled. They admitted me overnight for observation, but despite their best efforts, they couldn't pinpoint the exact cause of my symptoms. I was eventually sent home with medications and instructions to follow up with a specialist. The experience was unsettling, but after some time, I seemed to recover, and life moved on.

Fast forward to the birth of my son, and once again, that familiar sense of dread began to creep in. Something felt wrong. My feet were still swollen long after I expected them to return to normal. The doctors assured me it was just water retention, a common postpartum issue, and not something to worry about. But I couldn't shake the feeling that it was more than that. I explained to my doctor that when I lay down at night, I could feel a strange gurgling sensation in my lungs. Although my chest sounded clear during examinations, the doctor suggested it might be allergies or congestion and prescribed me medication.

But it wasn't just the gurgling in my lungs. My heart felt like it was racing at times, beating so fast it left me breathless. There were moments when it seemed to skip beats, leaving me lightheaded and anxious. I was constantly exhausted—far more than what I thought was normal after childbirth. Yes, I had just had a baby, and yes, I knew postpartum fatigue was real, but something in my gut told me this wasn't typical. Instead of getting better as my C-section scars healed, I felt weaker and more drained as the days passed.

Then one day, everything came crashing down. I was out shopping, doing something as simple as placing groceries on the counter, but it felt like I had just run a marathon. Sweat poured off me, drenching my clothes, and each step I took felt labored, like I couldn't get enough air into my lungs. By the time I got home, climbing the stairs felt impossible. Each step was a monumental effort, and I was gasping for breath. That's when I knew—I couldn't ignore this any longer. Something was seriously wrong, and it was time to head to the emergency room.

5

The Diagnosis

At the emergency room, I was given an EKG, blood tests, and other examinations. I thought maybe I was just exhausted from being a new mother. But then the doctor came in and told me something I will never forget: "Your results show that you're in heart failure." I was shocked. How could this happen?

The doctor explained that my heart wasn't working as it should, and the fluid in my body was backing up into my organs and lungs. That's why I couldn't breathe, and why my legs were so swollen. The fluid had started to affect my kidneys as well. I was immediately admitted and put on intravenous Lasix to help flush the water out of my system. My head was spinning, but I knew I had to get better for my babies. I remember being placed on Lasix intravenously and the nurse having to measure my urine every time I went which felt like every ten minutes. I continued this way for a few hours until I felt like I had no more liquid to be removed from my body.

I sat in that exam room feeling confused, depressed, anxious and overwhelmed. I did not know what to think or how to feel really, my world was spinning. What did this mean for me, for my family, for my babies? Would I get better, would my heart heal? Why was this happening to me? These were just a few thoughts going through my head. I was in disbelief, "heart failure"? I just couldn't get it out of my head. Streams of tears flowed down my face as I was dreading the worst, while also missing my children and not knowing what the near future held for me.

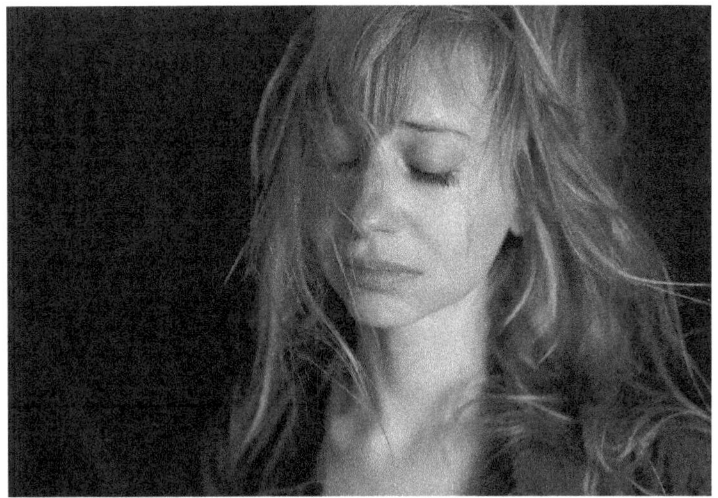

6

The Road to Recovery

The days following my diagnosis were a whirlwind of tests to determine just how severe my heart failure was. The results were devastating—my heart was functioning at a dangerously low level. I cried. I prayed. More than anything, I ached to be with my children. But deep down, I knew I had to fight, not just for them, but for myself.

The doctors prescribed multiple medications to strengthen my heart, but one of the hardest realities I faced was that I could no longer breastfeed my son. The very medications that were keeping me alive were unsafe for him, and that realization broke my heart.

My time in the hospital, though necessary, felt isolating. With COVID-19 at its peak, the hospital was on high alert. I was allowed only one visitor per day, which was a small comfort but still left me feeling lonely. To pass the time and take my mind off my health, I caught up on TV shows—something I wouldn't normally have the time for while caring for my little ones. I also listened to soothing music to keep myself calm and would walk the hospital hallways with my mask on, staring out at the garden and praying for my health to return.

After a week in the hospital, I was discharged. But my journey toward recovery had only just begun. I was put on a strict regimen that included severely limiting my water and salt intake to prevent fluid buildup. I was restricted to no more than six glasses of liquid a day—whether it was tea, coffee, juice, or even water-rich fruits. Every morning, I had to check my weight and blood pressure. If my weight increased by more than five pounds overnight, it was a dangerous sign that my body was retaining fluid, and I had to act fast.

For the next five months, I rigorously followed this routine, sticking closely to my diet and medication. It wasn't easy, but eventually, I went for another heart scan. To my immense relief, my heart function had improved. While I still had a small leaky valve that required ongoing monitoring, hearing that I had made it through the worst was overwhelming. I had been given a second chance—to live, to be there for my children, and to finally let go of the constant fear that my heart might fail me.

One of the greatest comforts during this difficult time was the support system the hospital provided. Upon discharge, I was given access to a nurse hotline, which allowed me to call with any questions or concerns about my health. I was also provided with a wellness package that included a scale, blood pressure monitor, oxygen meter, and other essential tools. Each time I recorded my vitals, the data was automatically sent to the clinic overseeing my recovery. If anything seemed off, they would immediately reach out to me.

This safety net was a tremendous source of relief. It eased my anxiety and reassured me that I wasn't in this fight alone. That support, combined with my determination to recover, gave me the strength to push through one of the darkest and most challenging times in my life.

7

Awareness Can Save Lives

Throughout my recovery, I did extensive research on postpartum cardiomyopathy, and I was shocked by how rare this condition is, yet how deadly it can be. I read stories of women who didn't survive—women who mistook their symptoms for typical postpartum discomfort and didn't seek help until it was too late. One story that stayed with me was about a woman who passed away in her sleep, never getting the chance to watch her baby grow. I couldn't help but think of how heartbreaking it must have been for her family—to experience the joy of bringing a child into the world, only to have that joy stolen by this silent killer.

What surprised me even more was how little information is available on postpartum cardiomyopathy. It's not a condition that's commonly screened for in expectant or new mothers, and that lack of awareness is terrifying. I searched for stories of other mothers who had experienced this and learned about how some made it through such a nightmarish ordeal. One story I found was about a mother who, despite being diagnosed, chose to have more children. Sadly, her heart function declined with each pregnancy, and she had to be constantly monitored to ensure her heart was functioning well enough to survive childbirth. In cases like this, the heart may never fully recover, and each subsequent pregnancy can worsen the damage.

I also came across stories of women who now live with life-long heart issues, never regaining normal heart function. These mothers have to take multiple medications just to maintain their heart's ability to pump blood, and many are restricted to a strict water and salt intake for the rest of their lives.

I'm sharing my story to raise awareness about this condition because knowing the signs can save your life. As new mothers, we often put ourselves last, prioritizing our children. But we must take care of our health so we can be there for them. If something doesn't feel right, trust your instincts and seek help. It could make all the difference.

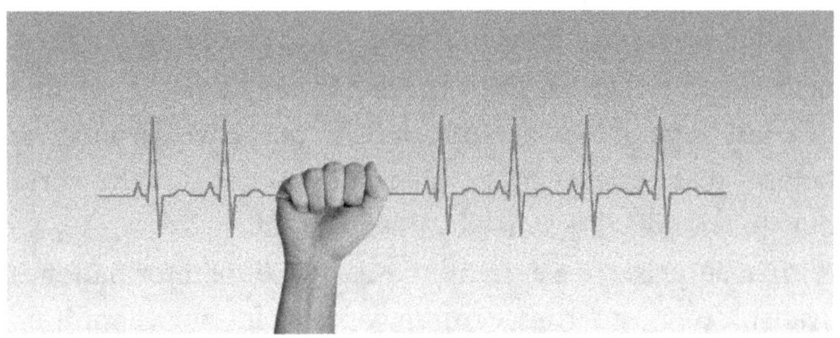

8

Conclusion

I consider myself incredibly fortunate. I survived postpartum cardiomyopathy and emerged stronger on the other side. While I may never be able to have another child, I am deeply grateful for the two beautiful children I have. My life—and being present for them—is far more valuable than risking it for another pregnancy.

I've learned to live life one day at a time, cherishing every moment I have with my children, watching them grow into the wonderful individuals they are becoming. This experience has profoundly changed my outlook on life. I no longer take it for granted. Life can shift in an instant, and I've realized the importance of telling those I love how much they mean to me, visiting with family and friends, and pausing to appreciate the simple beauty around us—the moon, the stars, and even just the feel of a deep breath in and out.

I've come to value these small moments and understand how quickly everything can change.

If my story can help even one mother recognize the signs and seek help, then sharing it was worthwhile. Peripartum/postpa rtum cardiomyopathy may be rare, but it is very real—and it is a silent killer. Be vigilant, stay aware, and always trust your instincts. It could save your life.

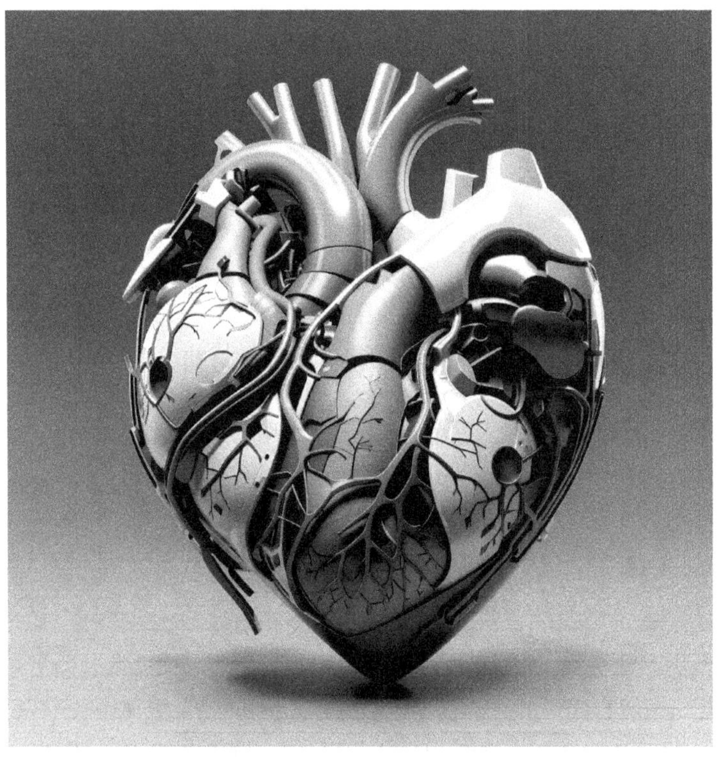

9

Postpartum Cardiomyopathy: What You Need to Know:

Definition

Peripartum cardiomyopathy (PPCM), also known as postpartum cardiomyopathy, is a rare form of heart failure that occurs in the final month of pregnancy or within five months after delivery. It weakens the heart's ability to pump blood and is often misdiagnosed as regular postpartum recovery.

Symptoms

- Shortness of breath
- Fatigue
- Fluid retention causing swollen ankles or feet
- Chest pain or tightness
- Heart palpitations

Here are a few important key facts on what to look out for whether you are a new mom, spouse or caregiver:

How a Person May Feel:

1. **Extreme Fatigue:** Beyond the usual tiredness associated with being a new mother, PPCM causes an overwhelming and unusual level of fatigue that makes even simple tasks exhausting.
2. **Shortness of Breath:** Many women report feeling out of breath, even when resting or performing light activities like walking or climbing stairs. This can sometimes be mistaken for postpartum recovery or lack of fitness after pregnancy.
3. **Swelling (Edema):** PPCM often causes swelling in the legs, ankles, and feet, which is common after pregnancy, but the swelling may also occur in the hands or abdomen and be more severe.
4. **Chest Pain or Discomfort:** Some women experience chest tightness or pressure, similar to the feeling of heartburn, but it can be more intense.

How a Person May Sound:

1. **Wheezing or Coughing:** The buildup of fluid in the lungs due to heart failure can cause a persistent cough or wheezing, especially when lying down.
2. **Labored Breathing:** Even when not physically exerting themselves, a person with PPCM might sound like they are struggling to breathe or catching their breath frequently.

How a Person May Act:

1. **Restlessness or Anxiety:** Many women feel increasingly anxious, agitated, or unable to settle down due to constant discomfort and difficulty breathing, which may be dismissed as stress from new motherhood.
2. **Difficulty with Physical Activity:** Someone with PPCM may avoid physical activities they would typically manage, like carrying their baby or walking around the house, due to rapid exhaustion or shortness of breath.

Recognizing these symptoms and seeking immediate medical attention is crucial, as PPCM can lead to life-threatening heart failure if left untreated.

If you experience any of these symptoms, seek medical attention immediately.

Thank you for taking the time to read my story. My hope in sharing this deeply personal journey is to raise awareness about postpartum cardiomyopathy and the very real dangers it poses to new mothers. This condition often goes undetected, its symptoms mistaken for the normal struggles of postpartum recovery. But by spreading knowledge and encouraging vigilance, I believe we can protect others from the silent and often deadly threat it carries.

If my experience can help even one mother recognize the signs and seek timely medical care, then this story has served its purpose. No woman should have to face this without the information and support she deserves. My goal is to ensure that all mothers, their families, and healthcare providers are equipped to recognize these subtle yet dangerous symptoms, so no one has to suffer in silence.

I sincerely hope that my journey will inspire you to take action, spread awareness, and empower others. Together, we can make a difference and save lives.

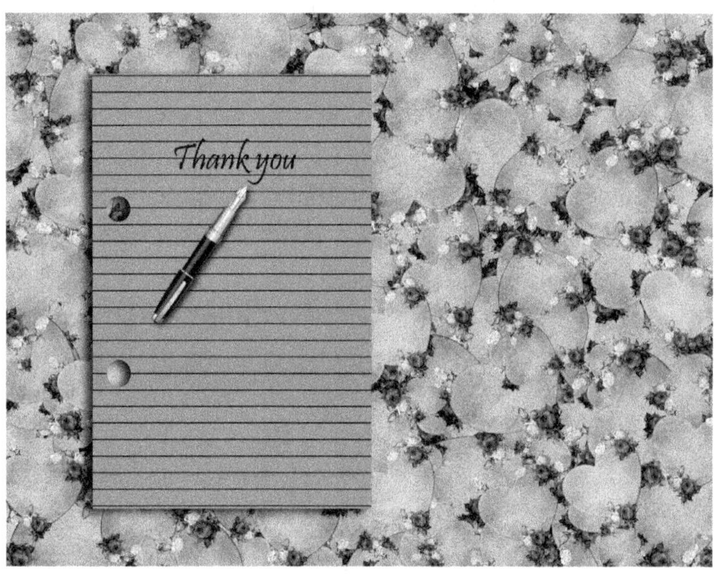